Coloring book for adults and kids human anatomy image for design

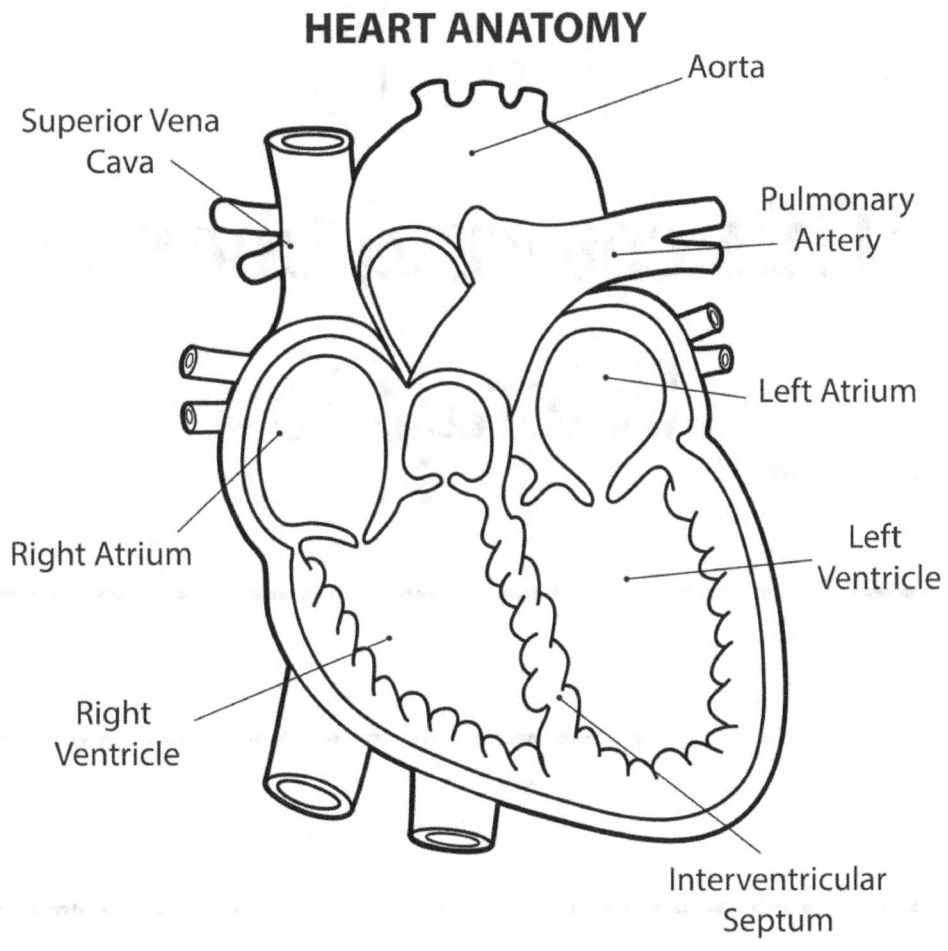

HEART ANATOMY

- Superior Vena Cava
- Aorta
- Pulmonary Artery
- Left Atrium
- Right Atrium
- Left Ventricle
- Right Ventricle
- Interventricular Septum

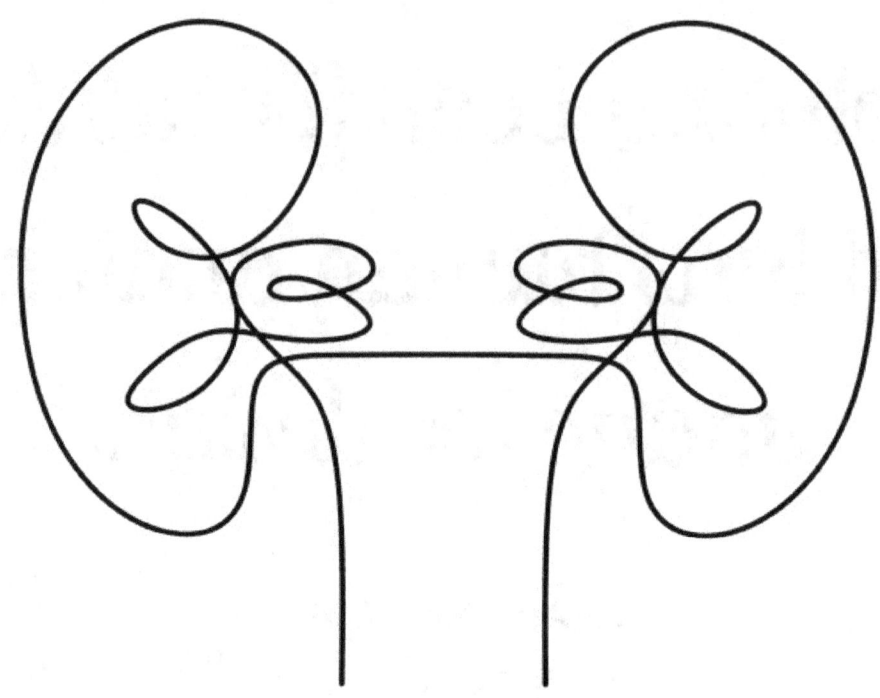

This coloring book is belongs to

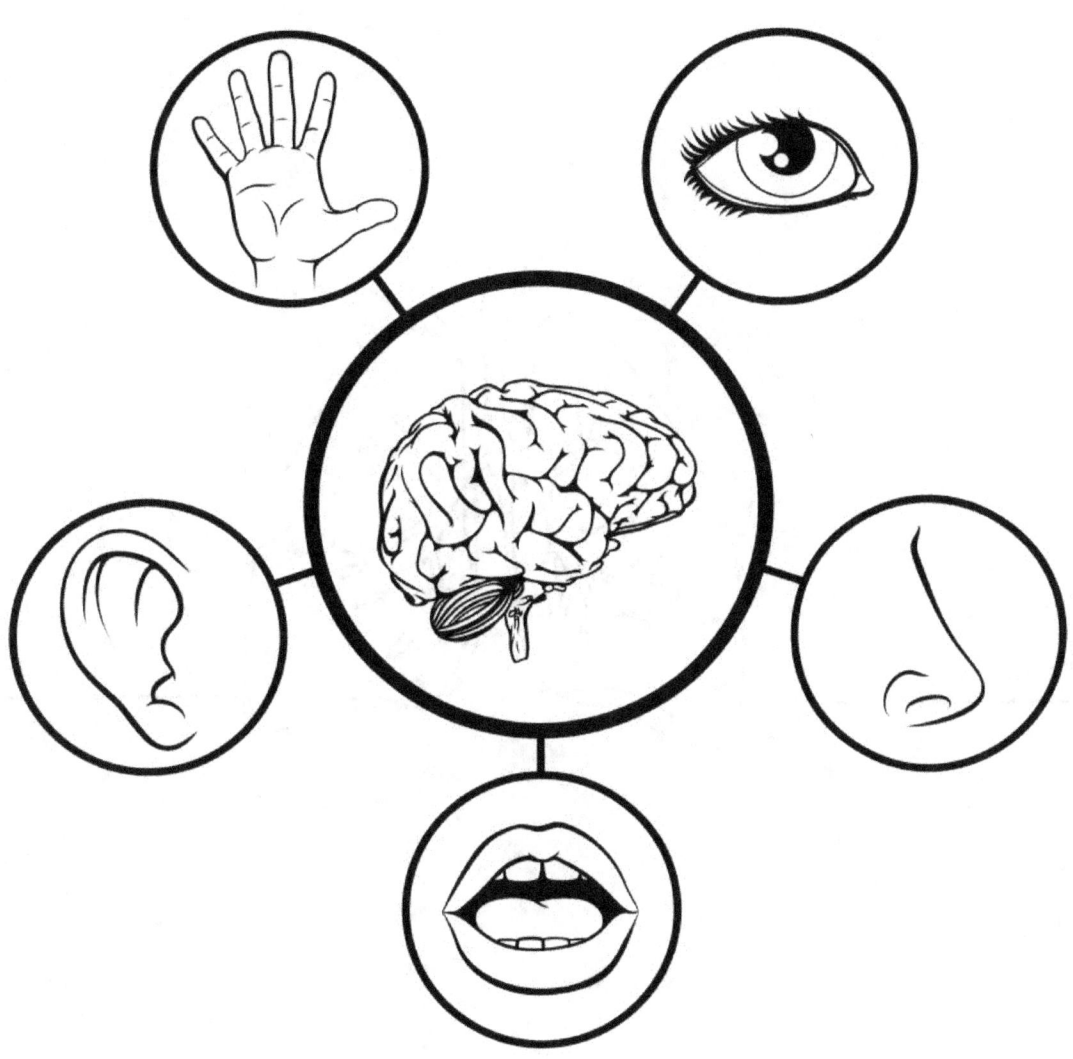

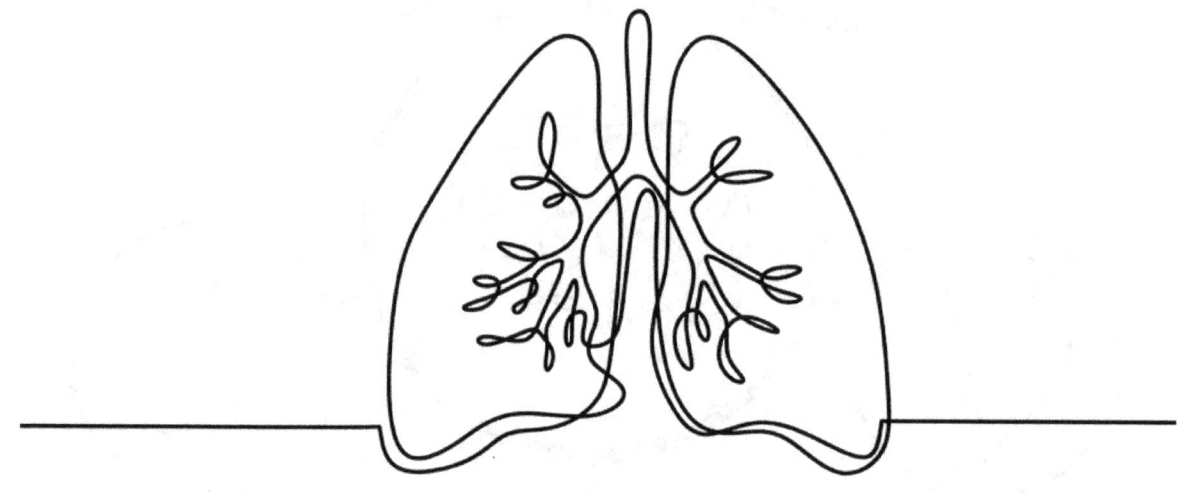

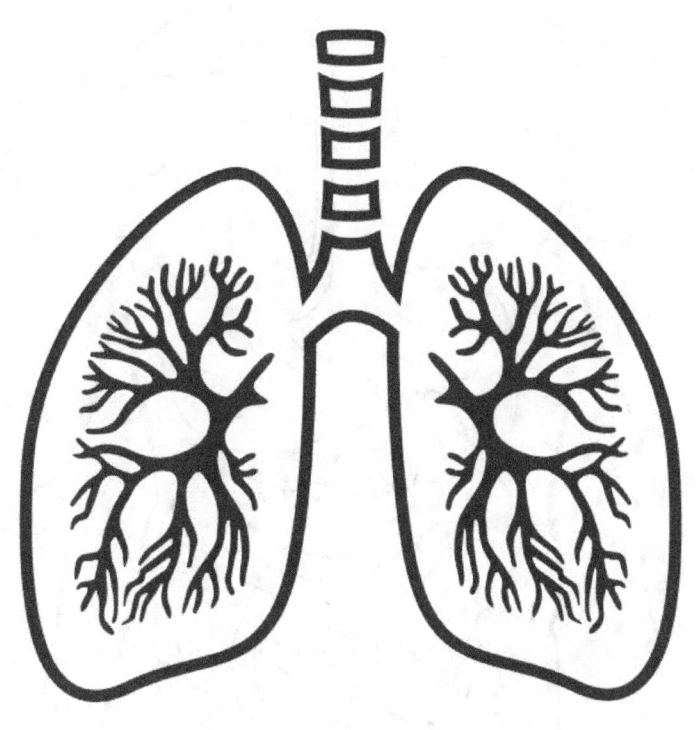

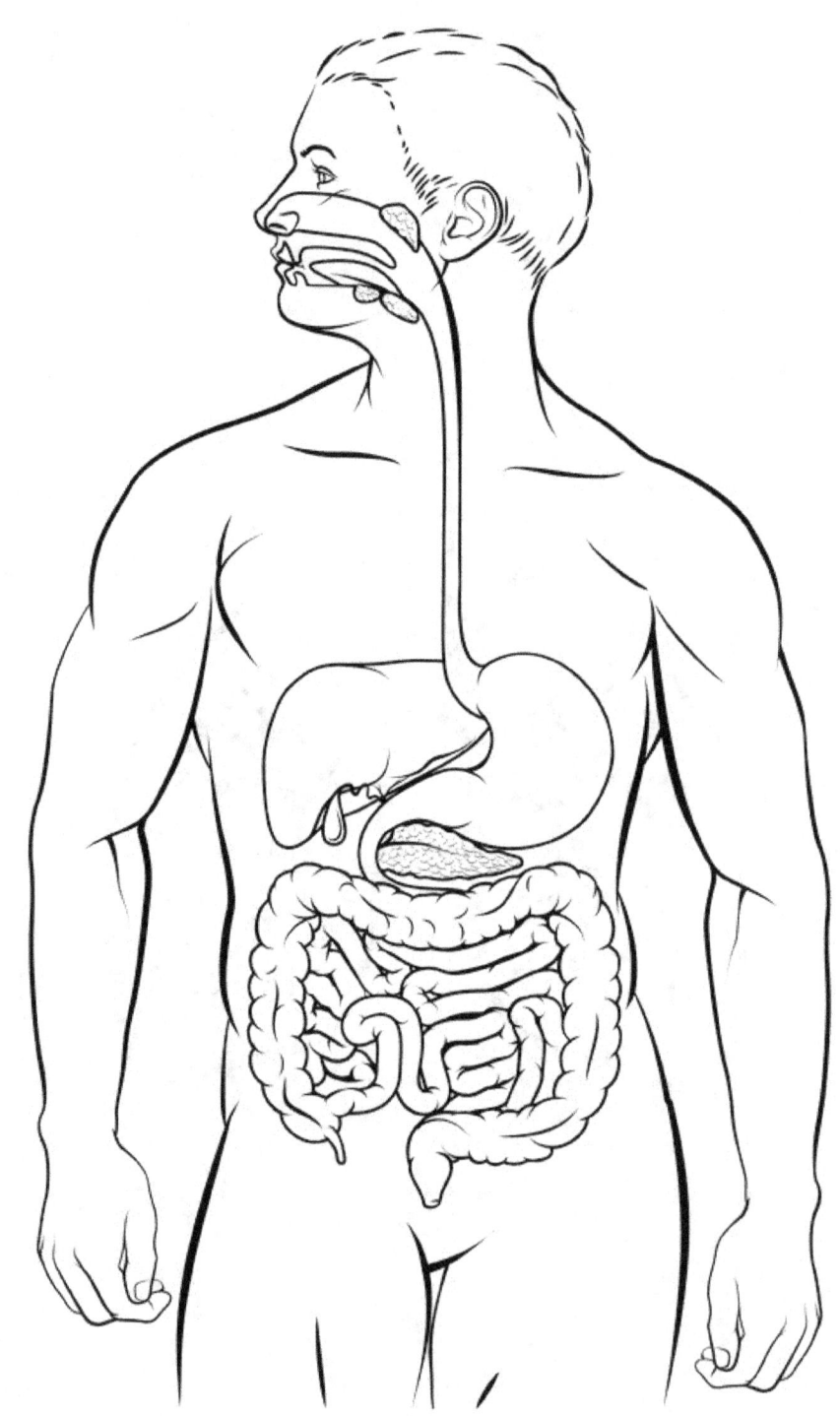

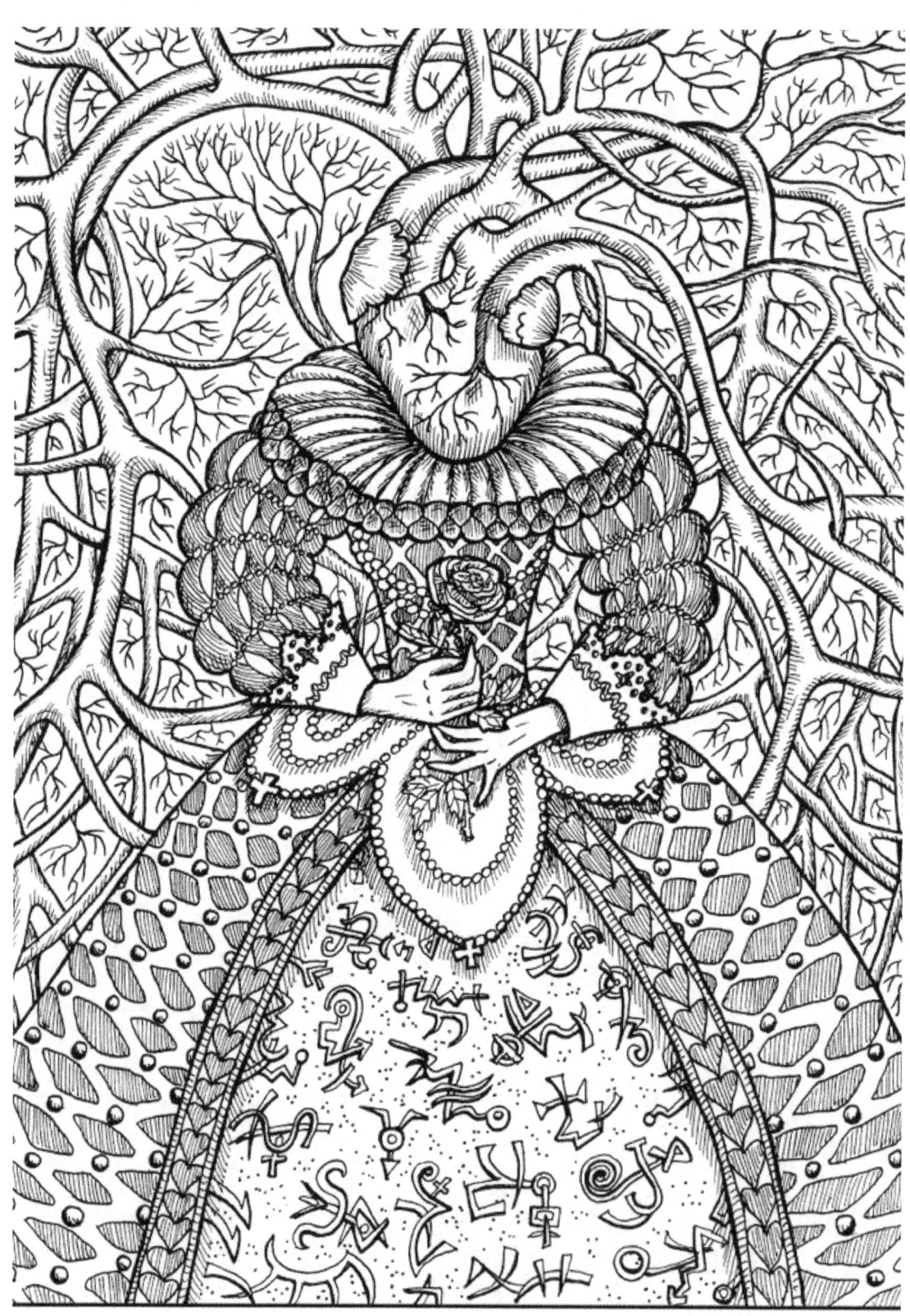

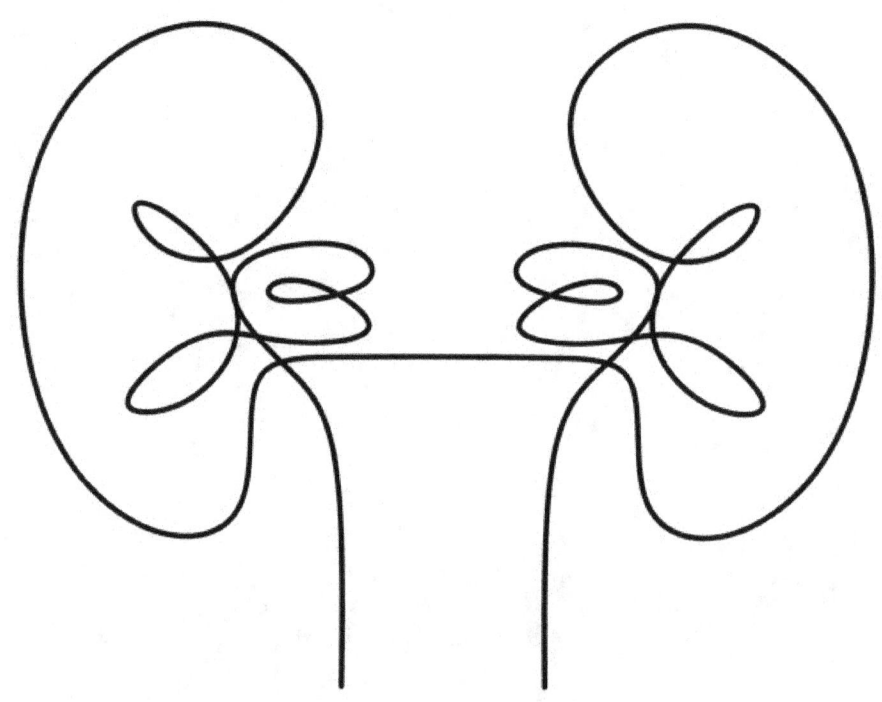

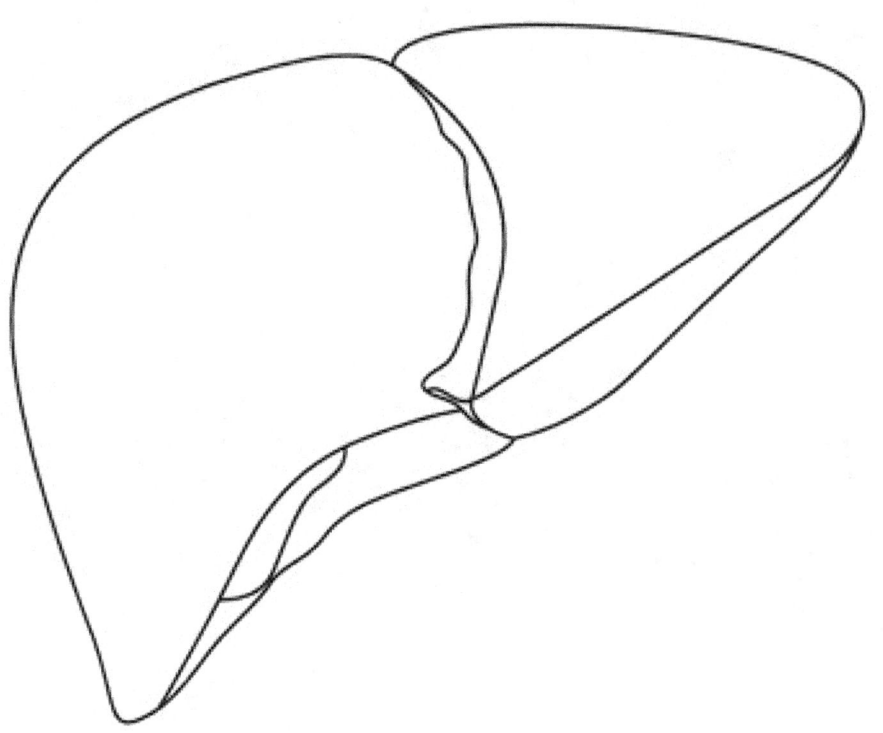

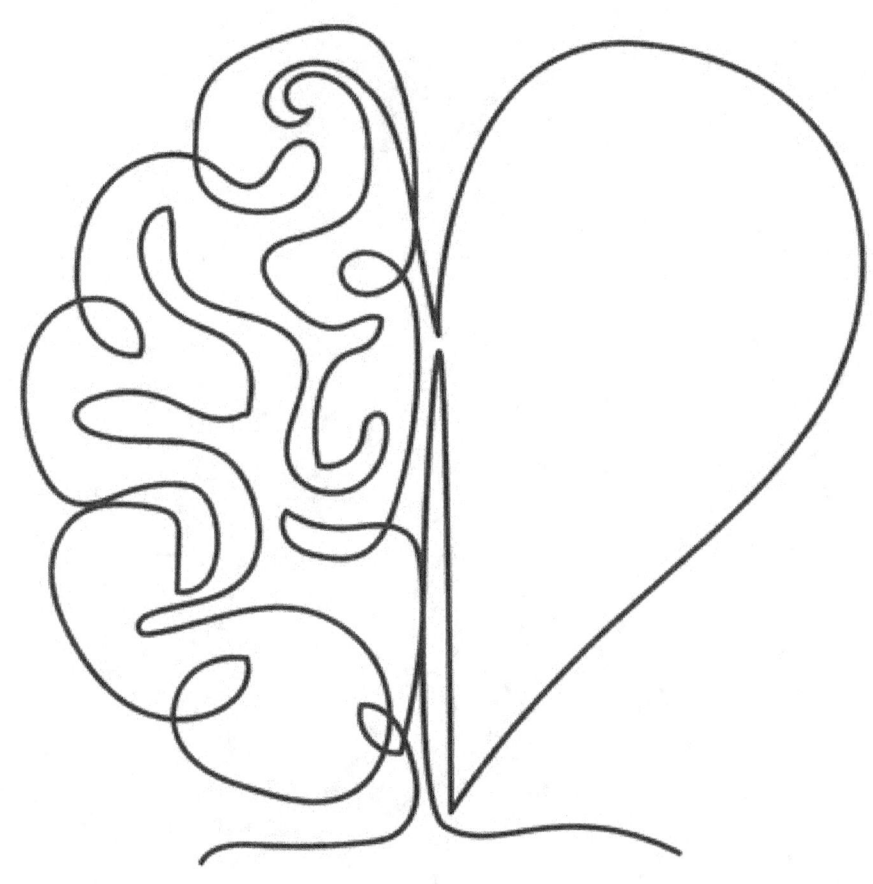

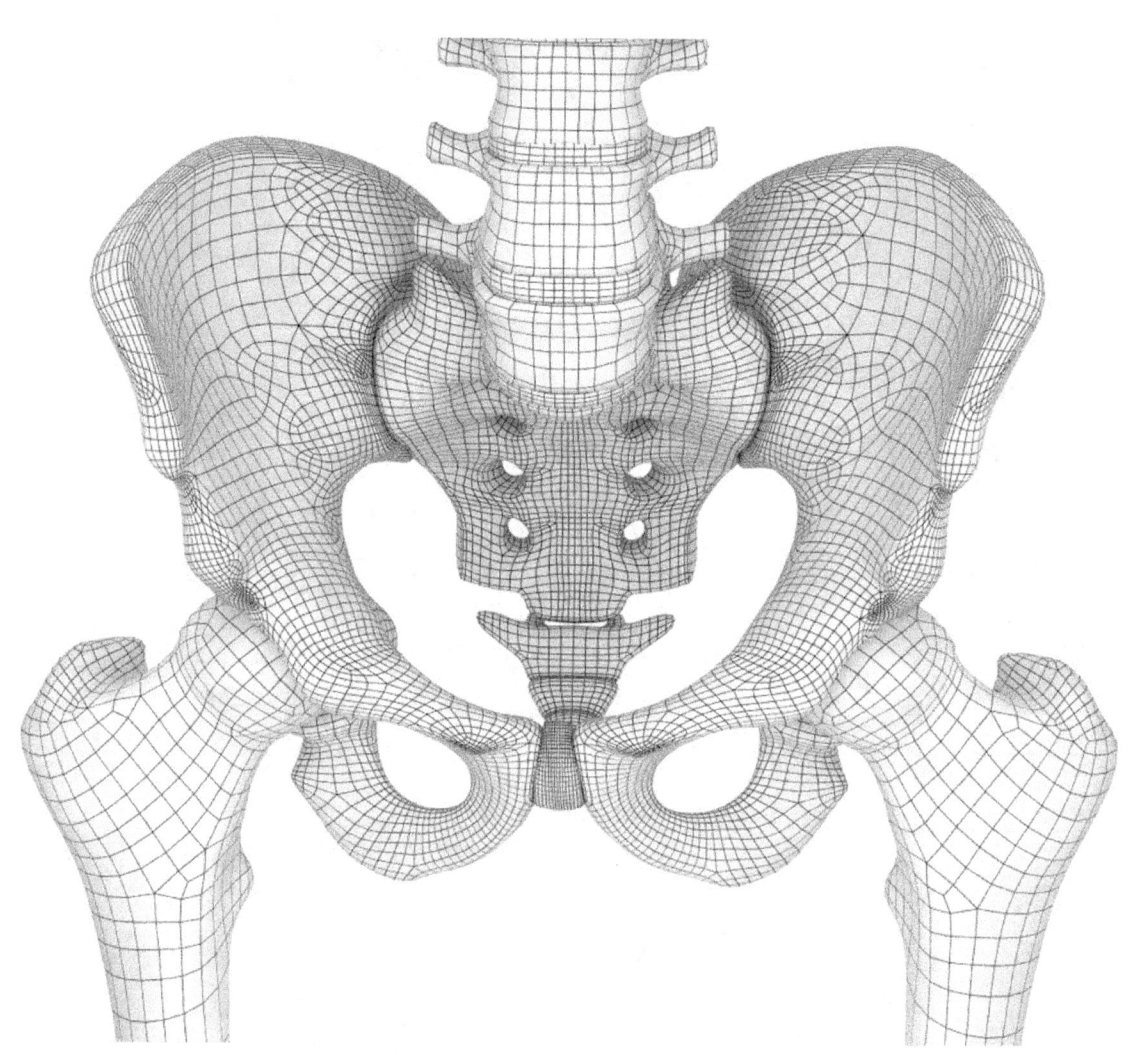

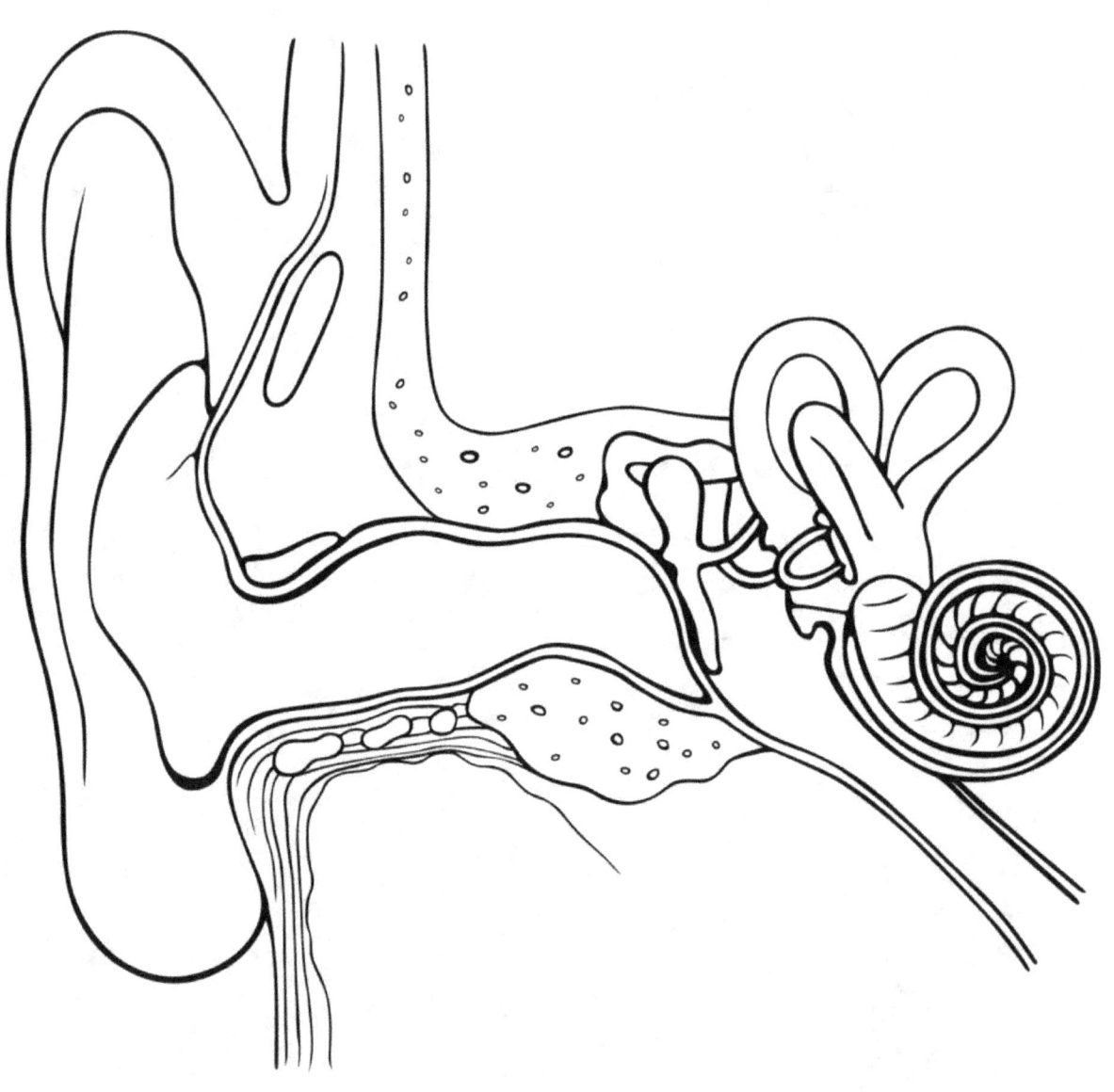

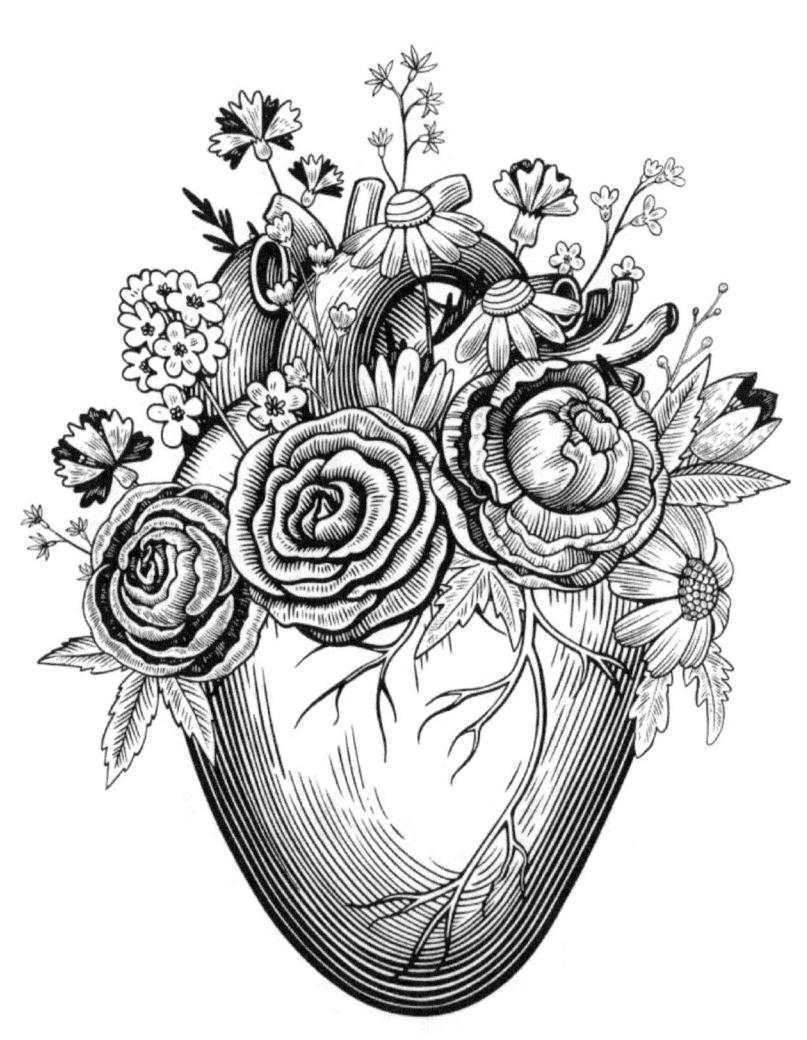

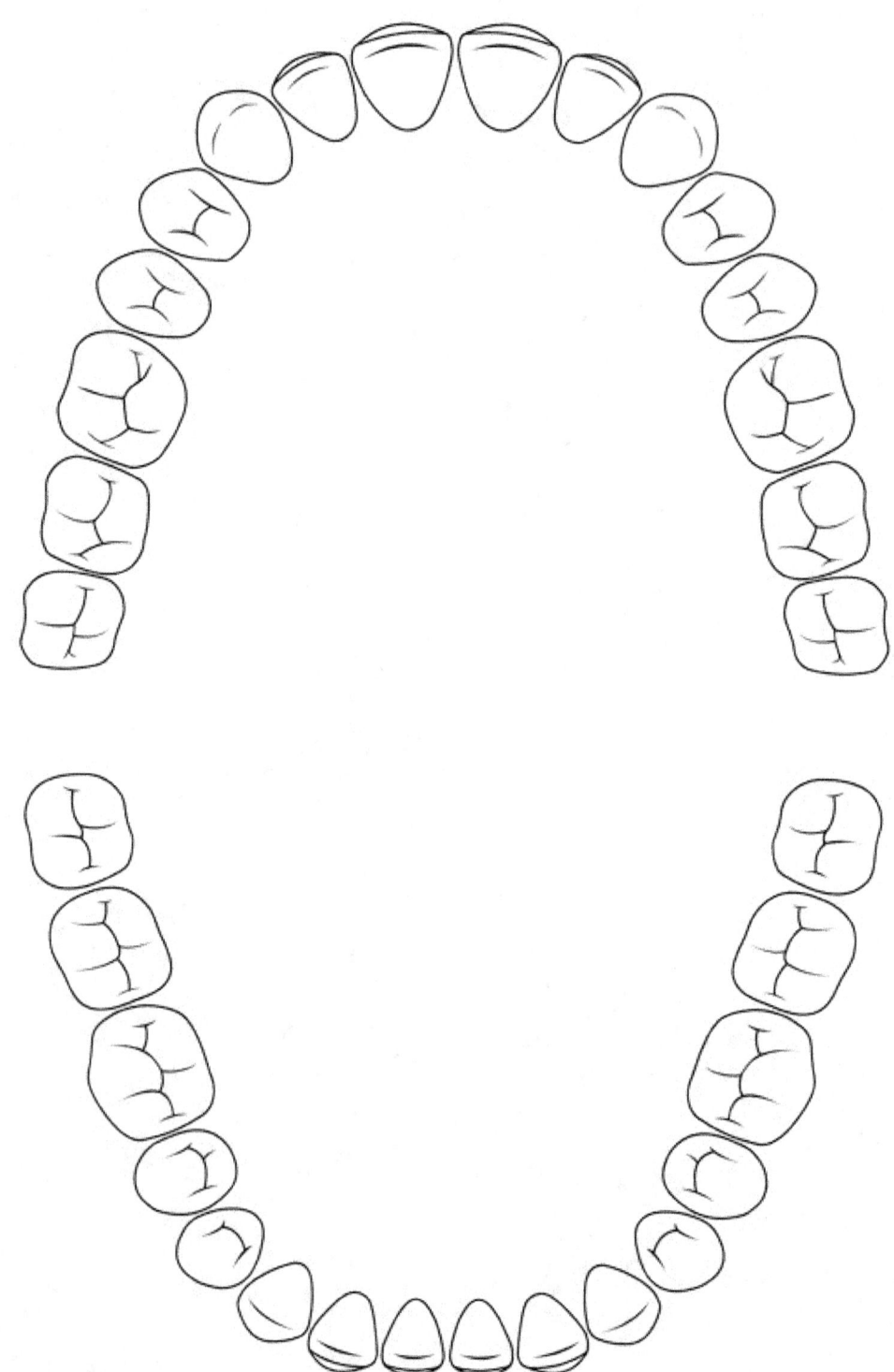

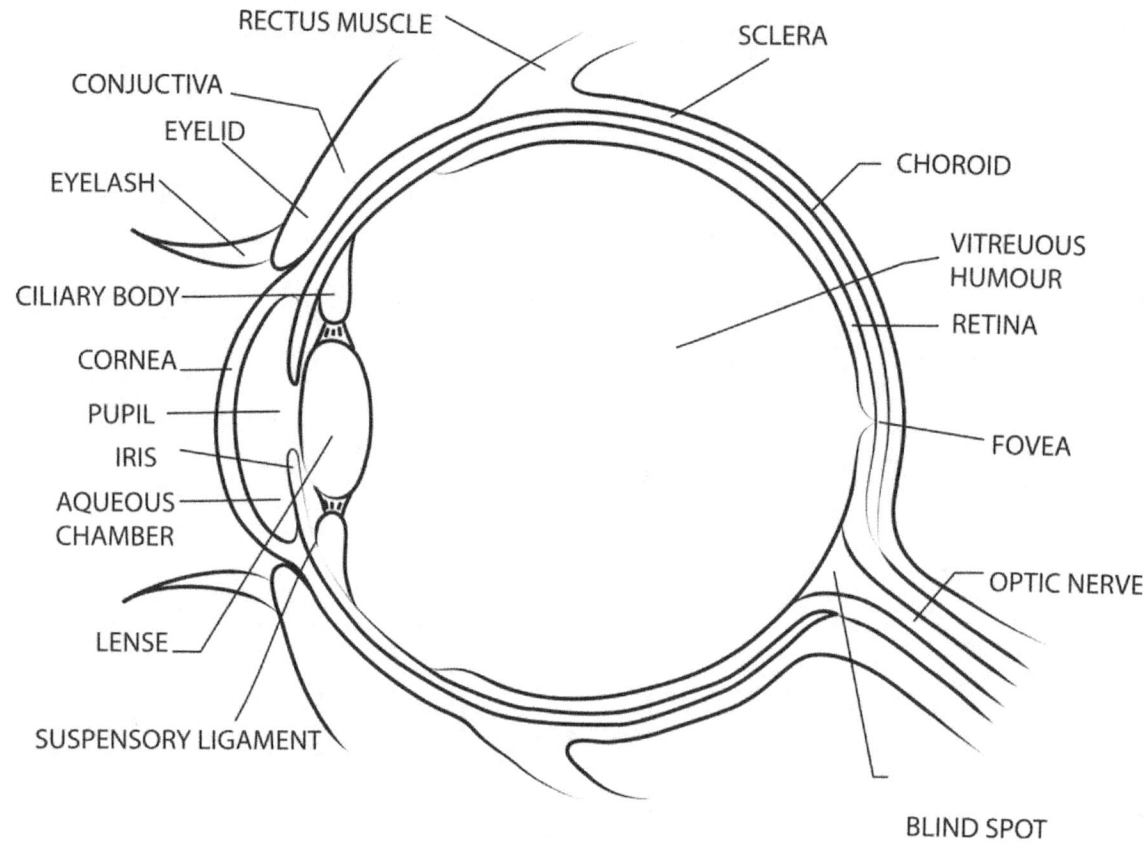

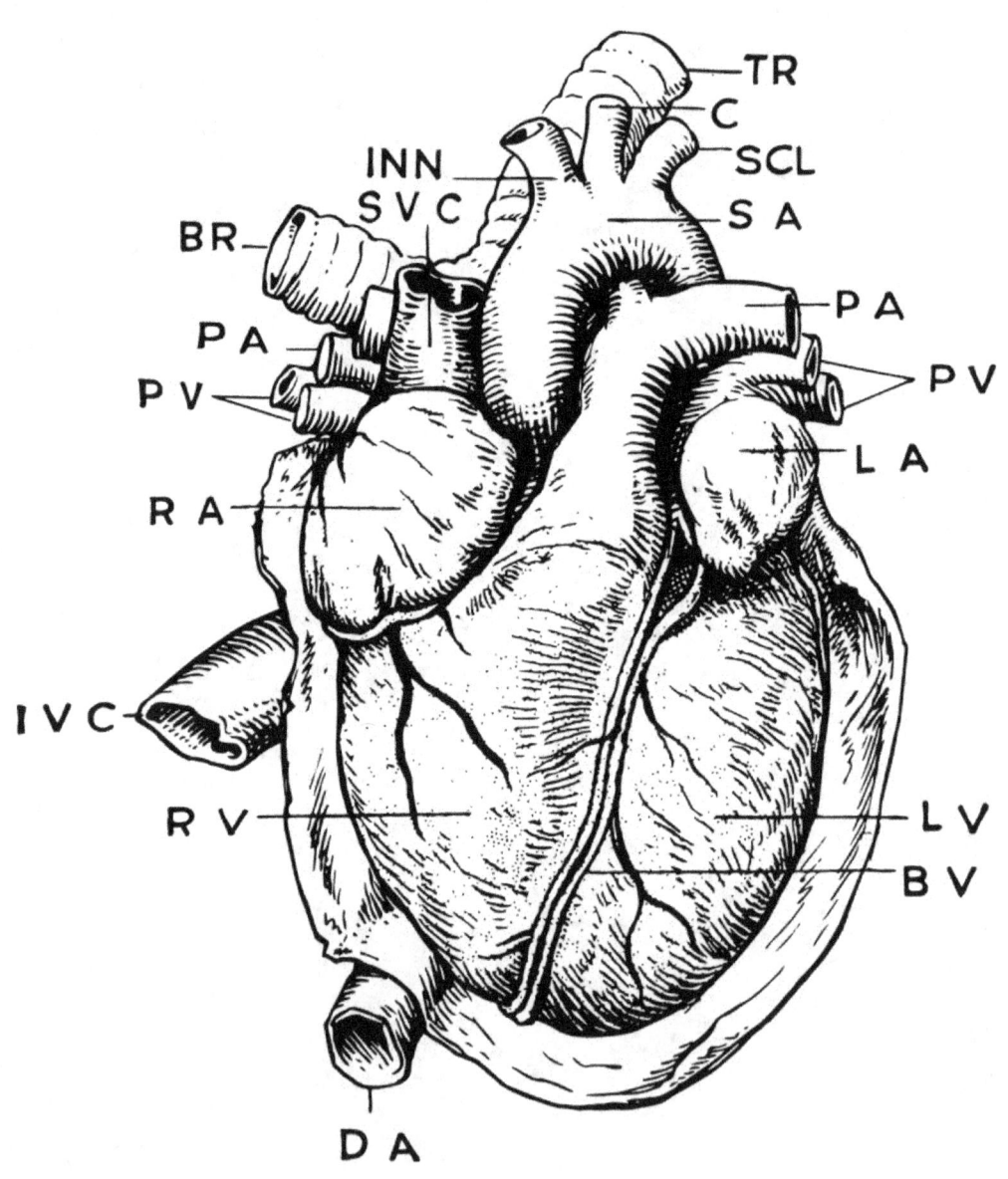

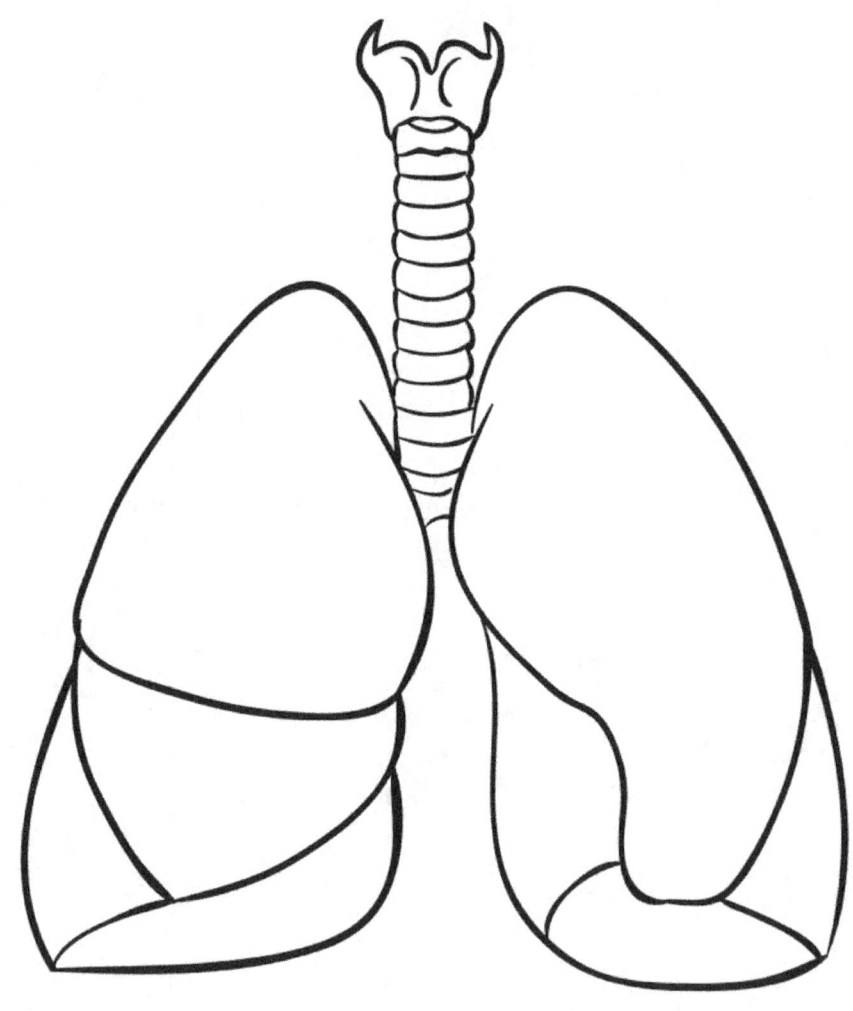

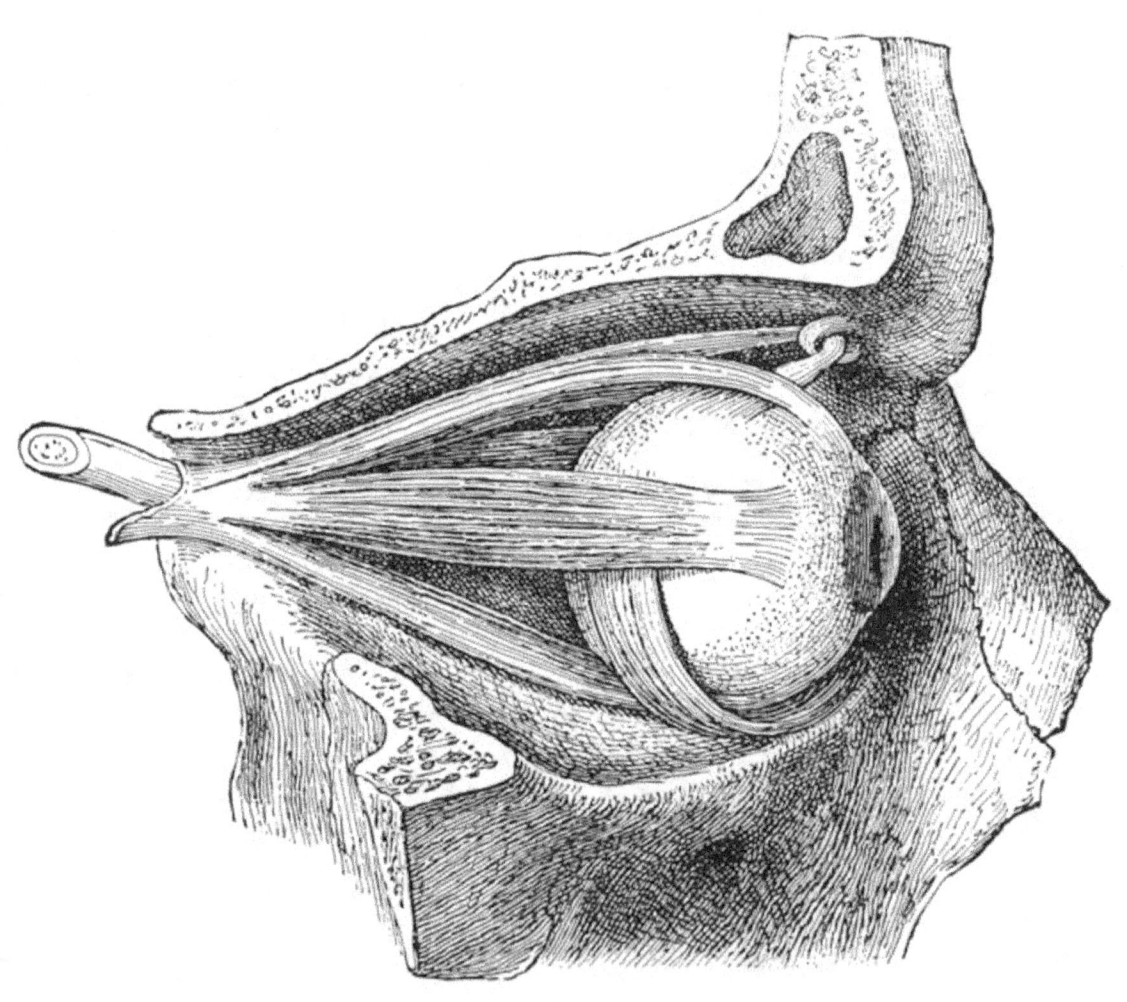

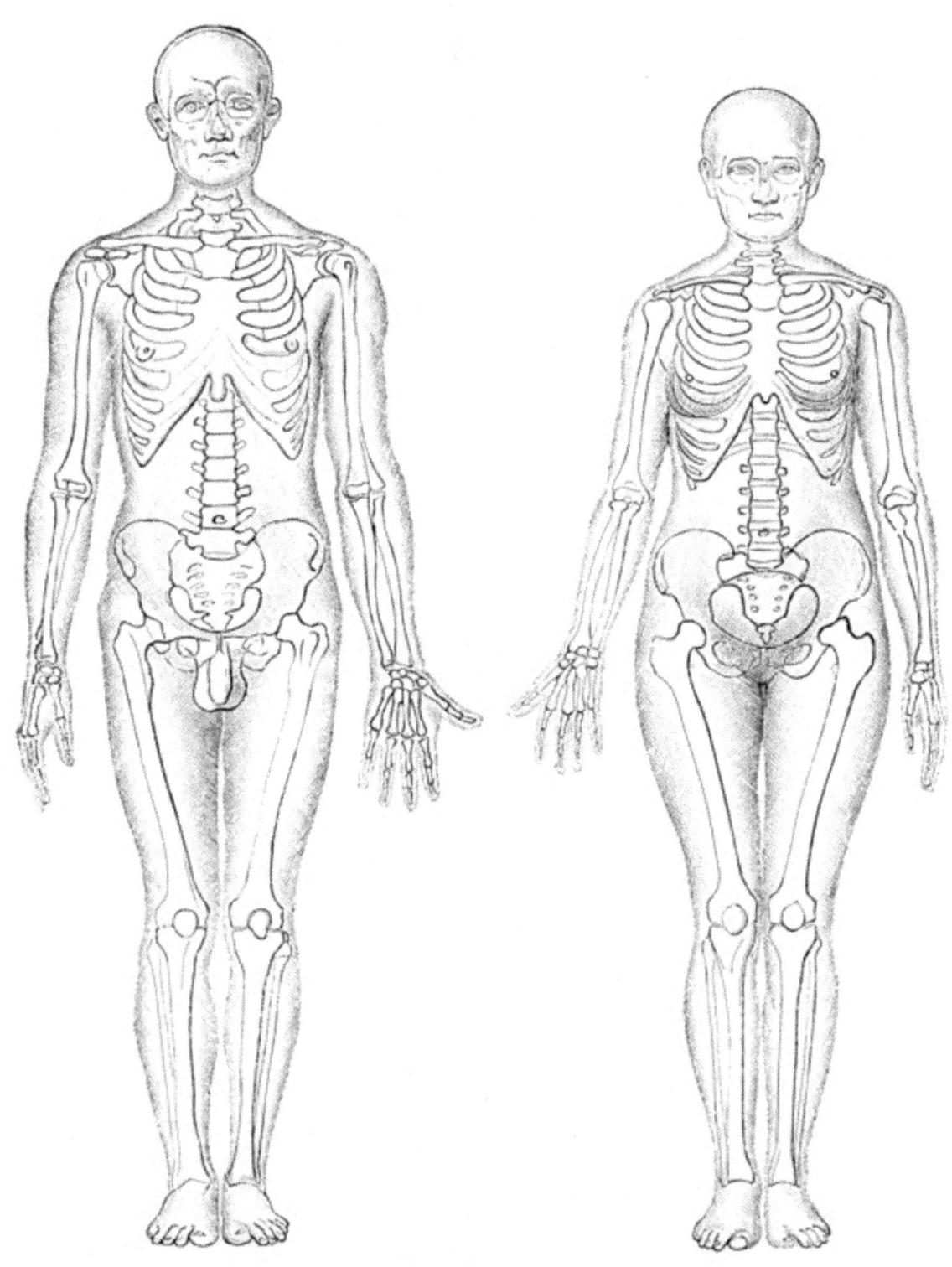

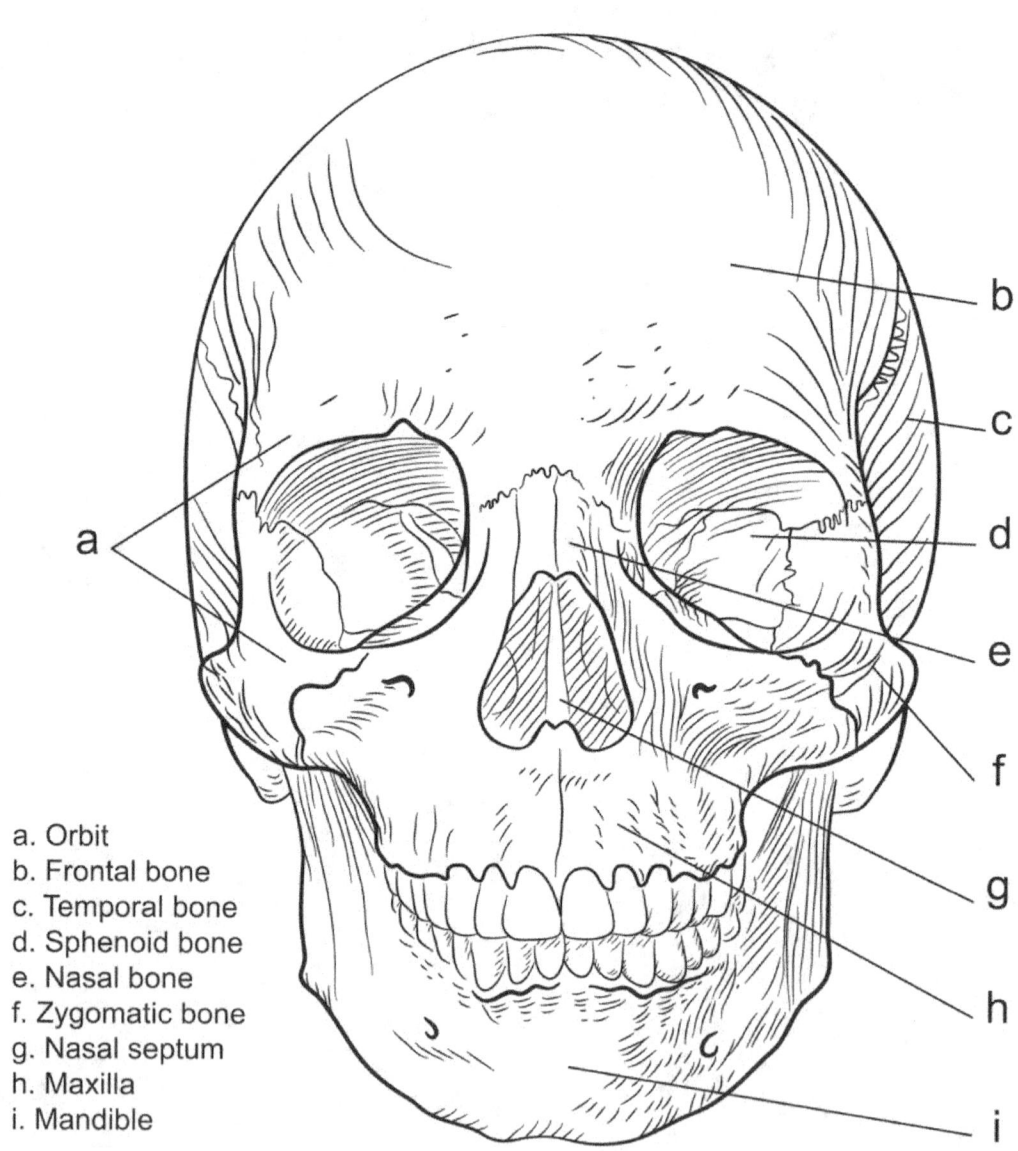

a. Orbit
b. Frontal bone
c. Temporal bone
d. Sphenoid bone
e. Nasal bone
f. Zygomatic bone
g. Nasal septum
h. Maxilla
i. Mandible

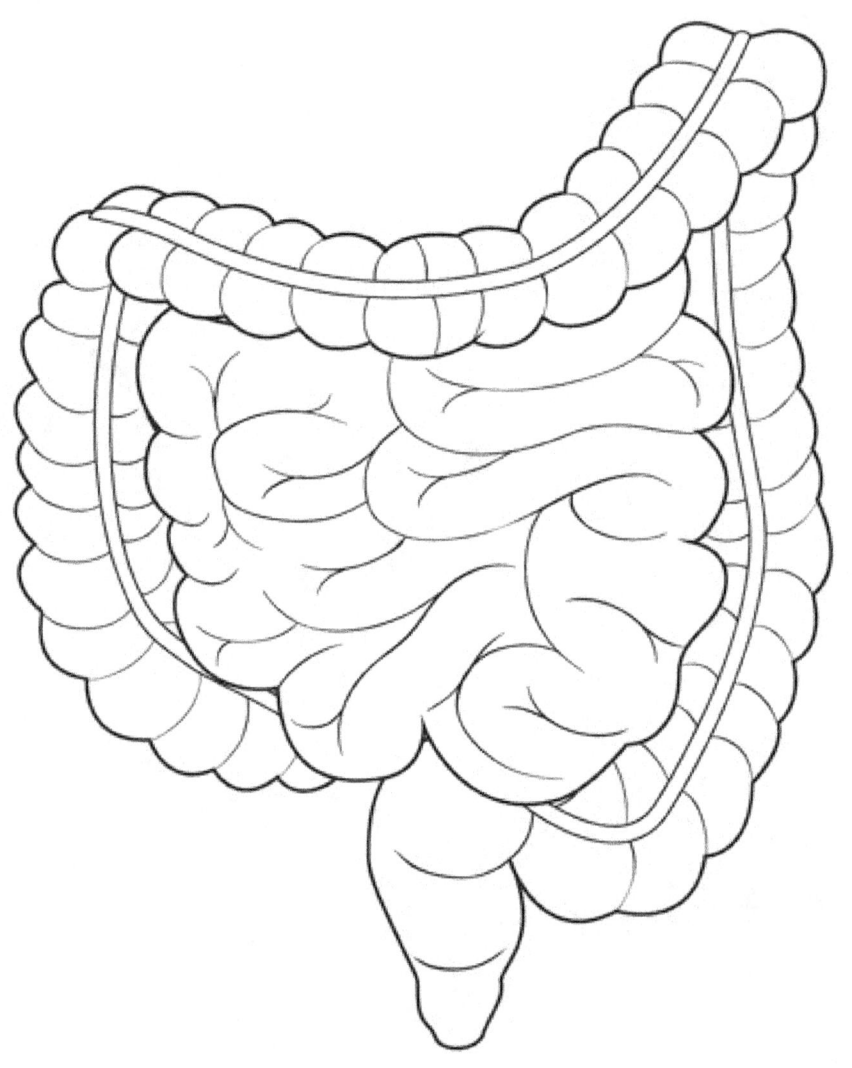

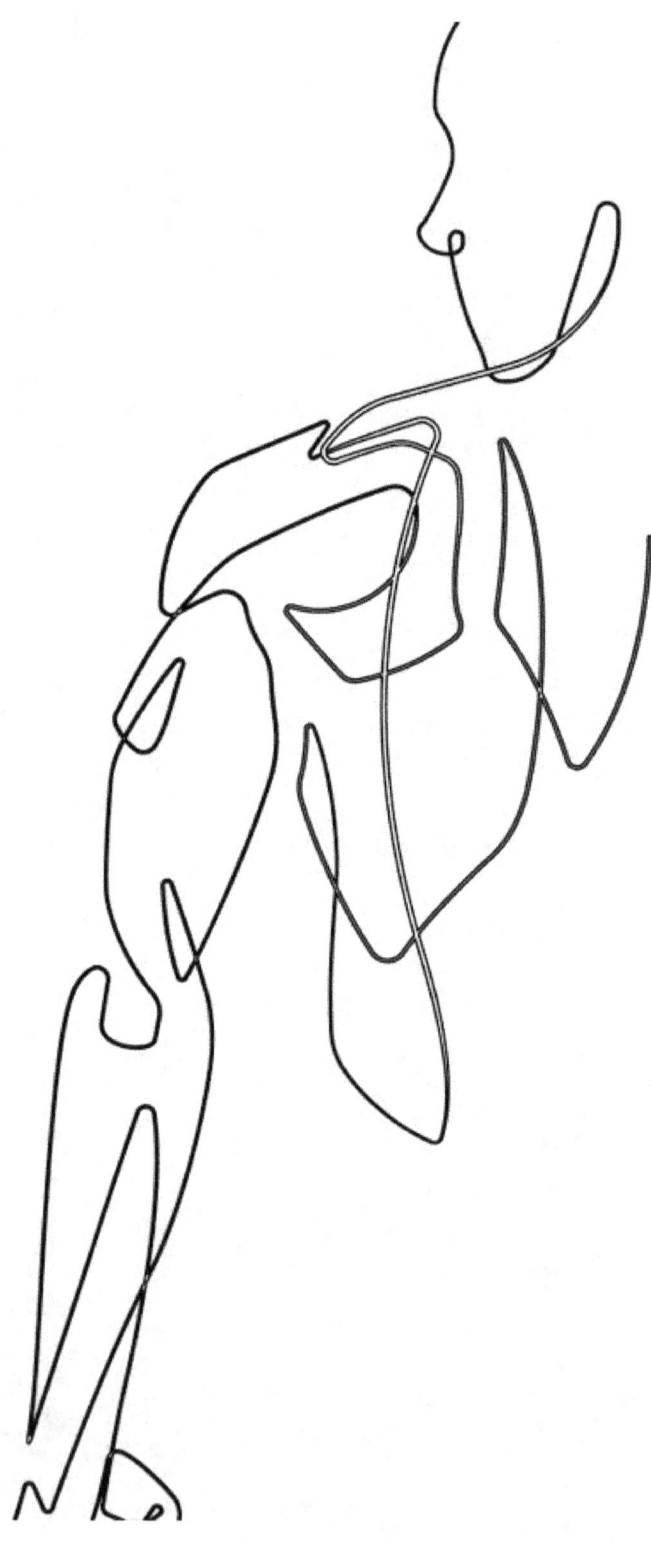

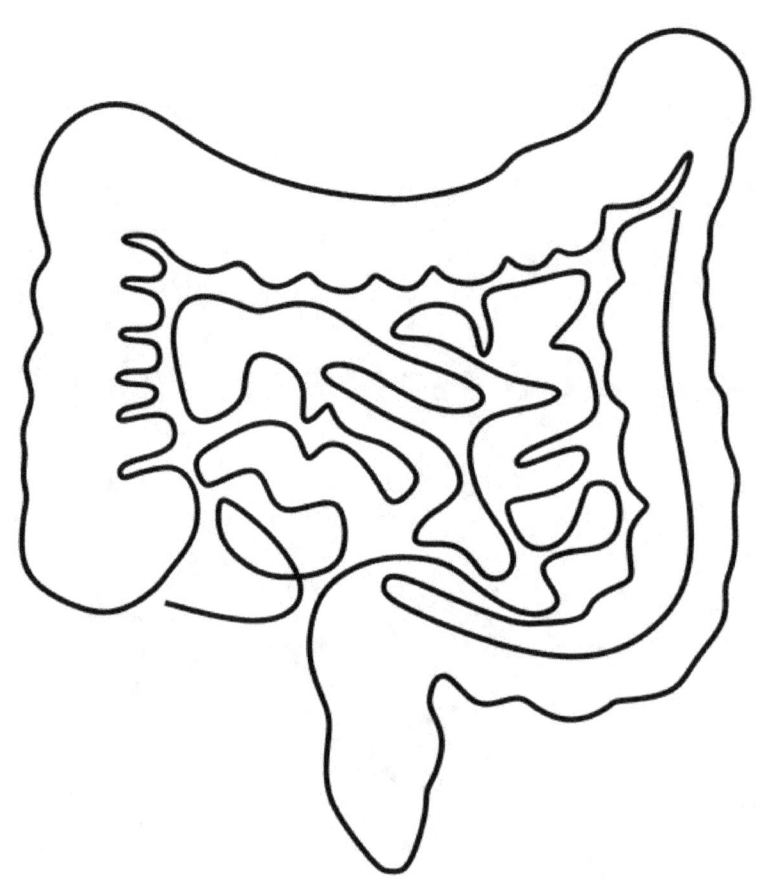

HEART ANATOMY

- Aorta
- Superior Vena Cava
- Pulmonary Artery
- Left Atrium
- Right Atrium
- Left Ventricle
- Right Ventricle
- Interventricular Septum

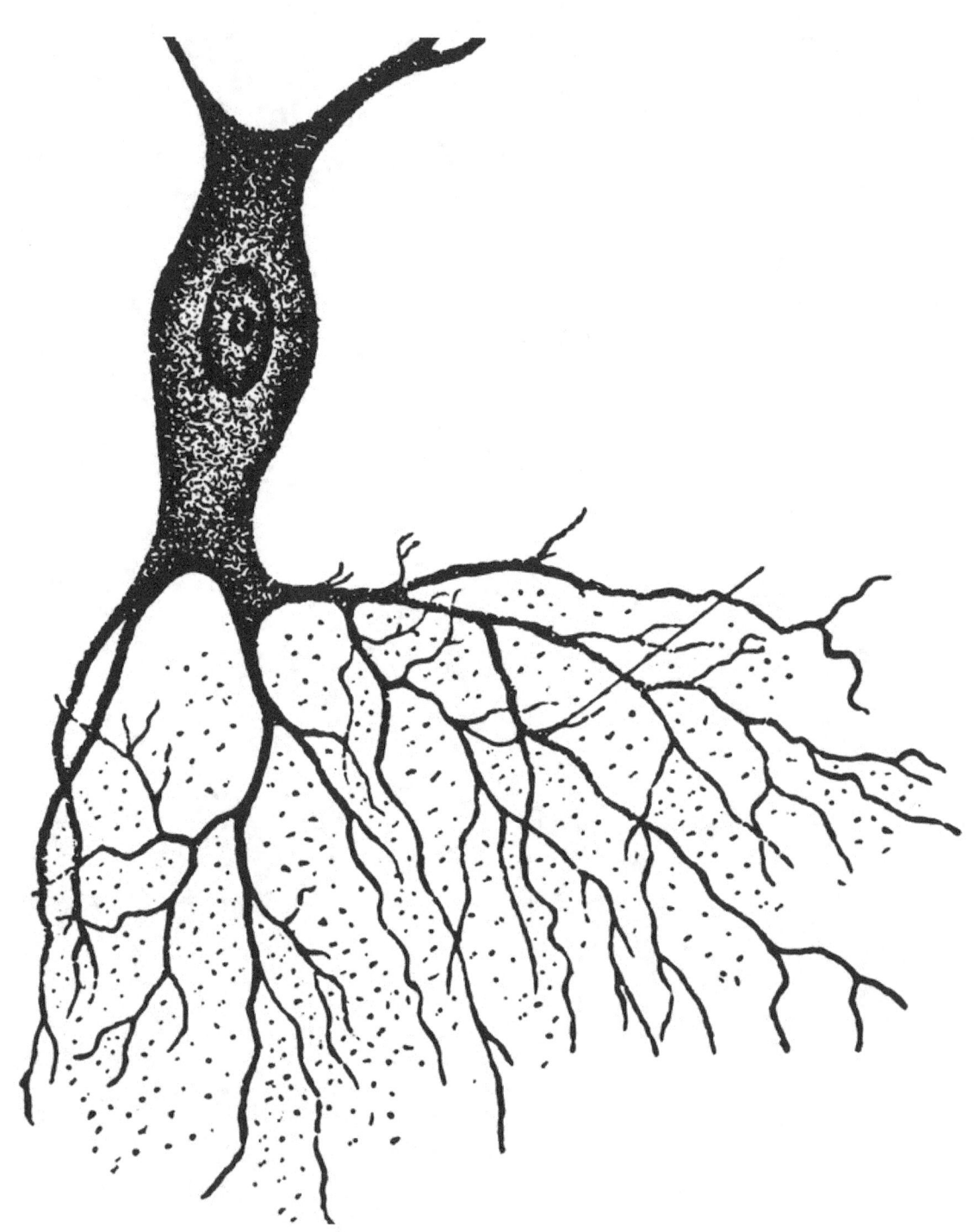

Human Skeletal System

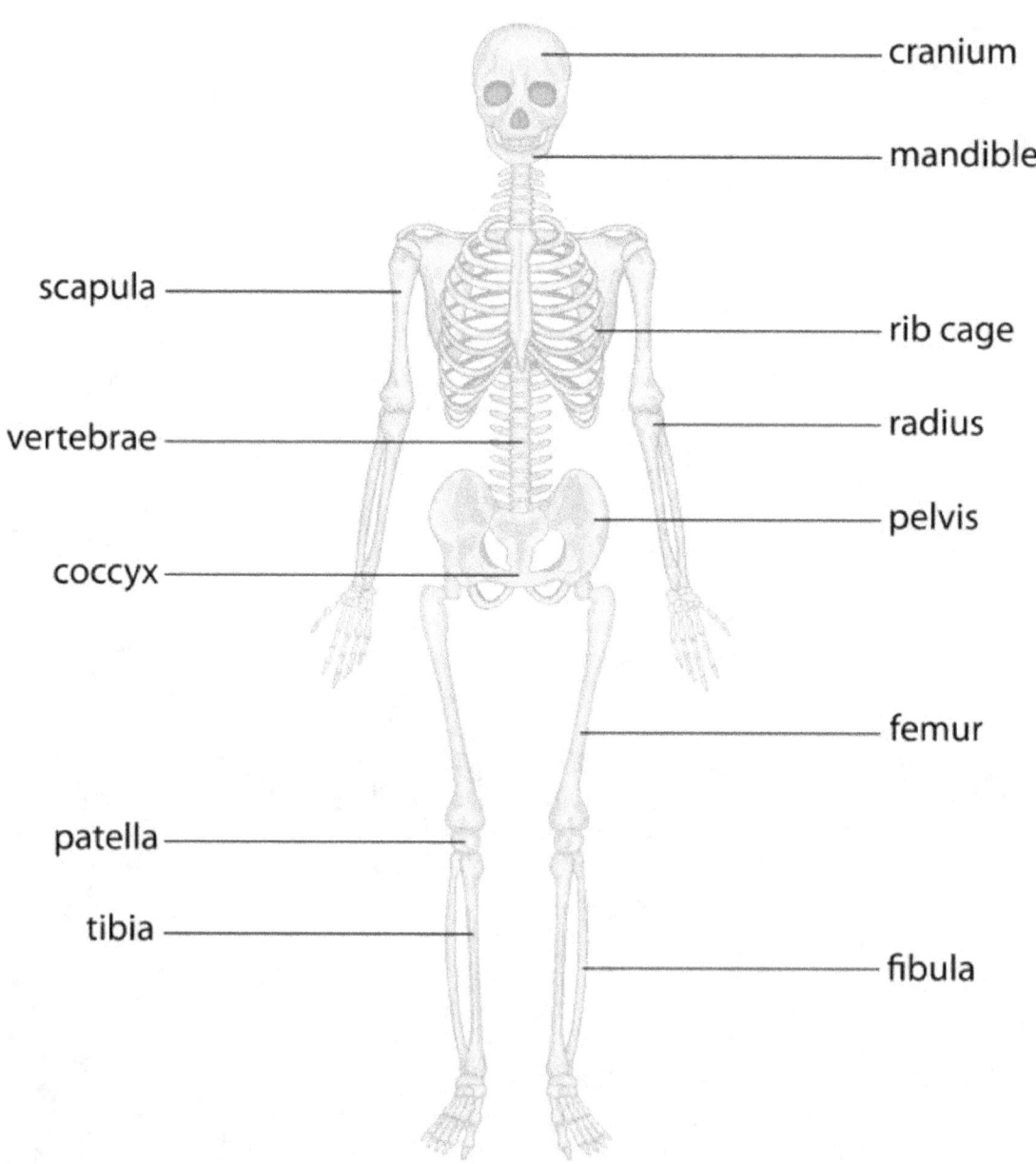

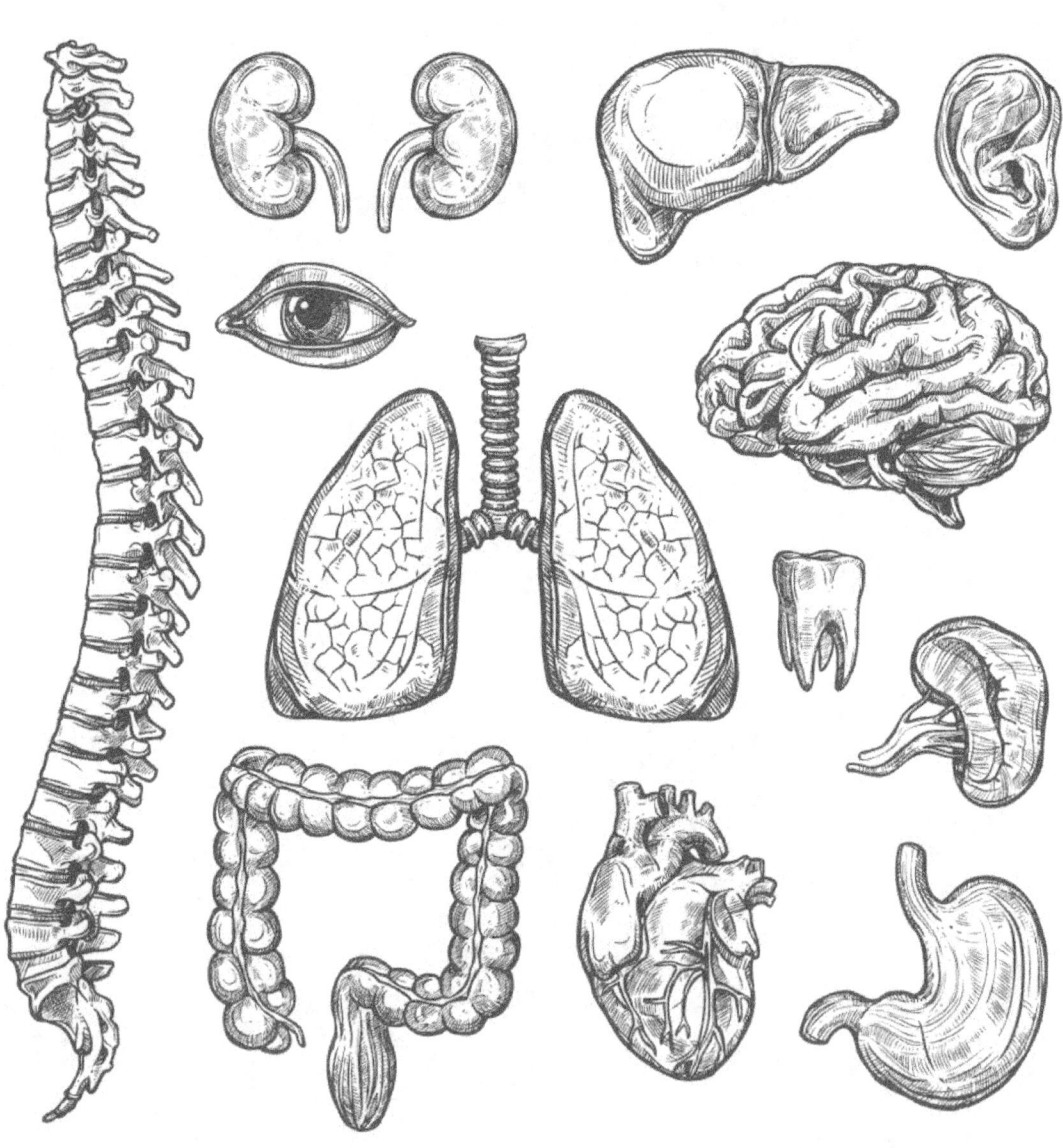

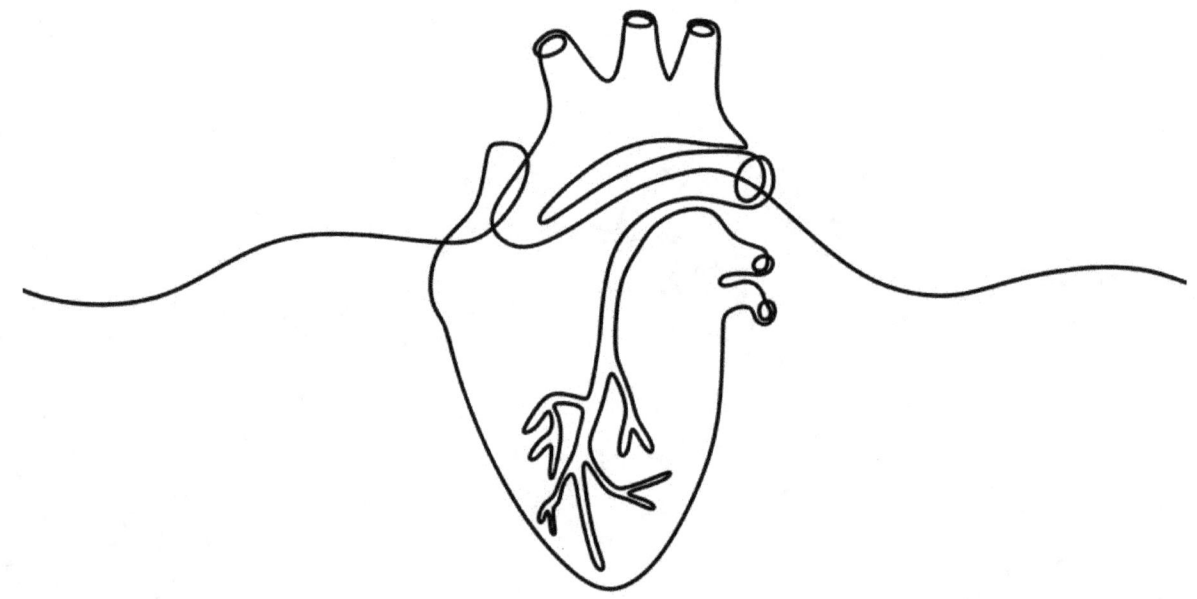

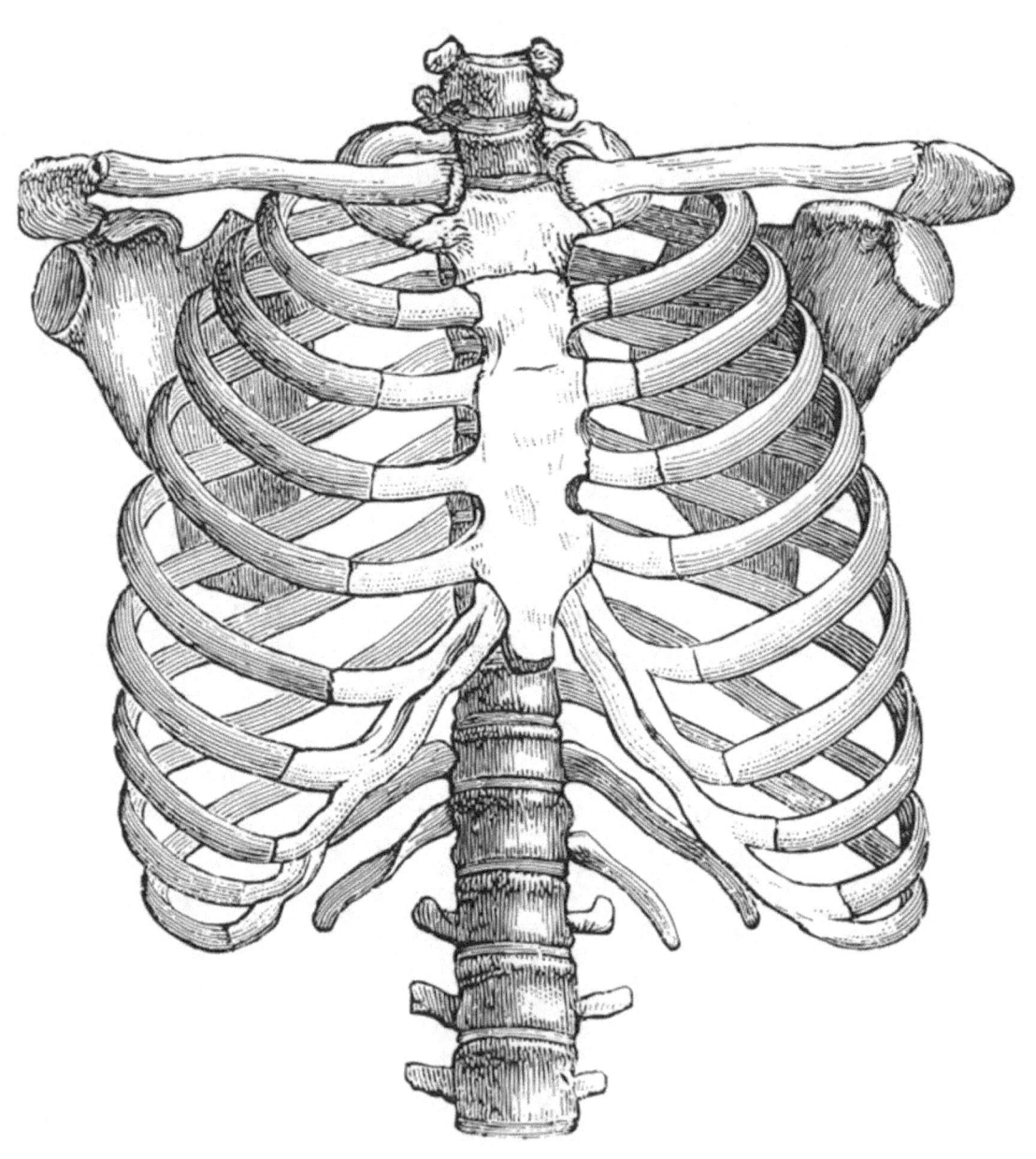

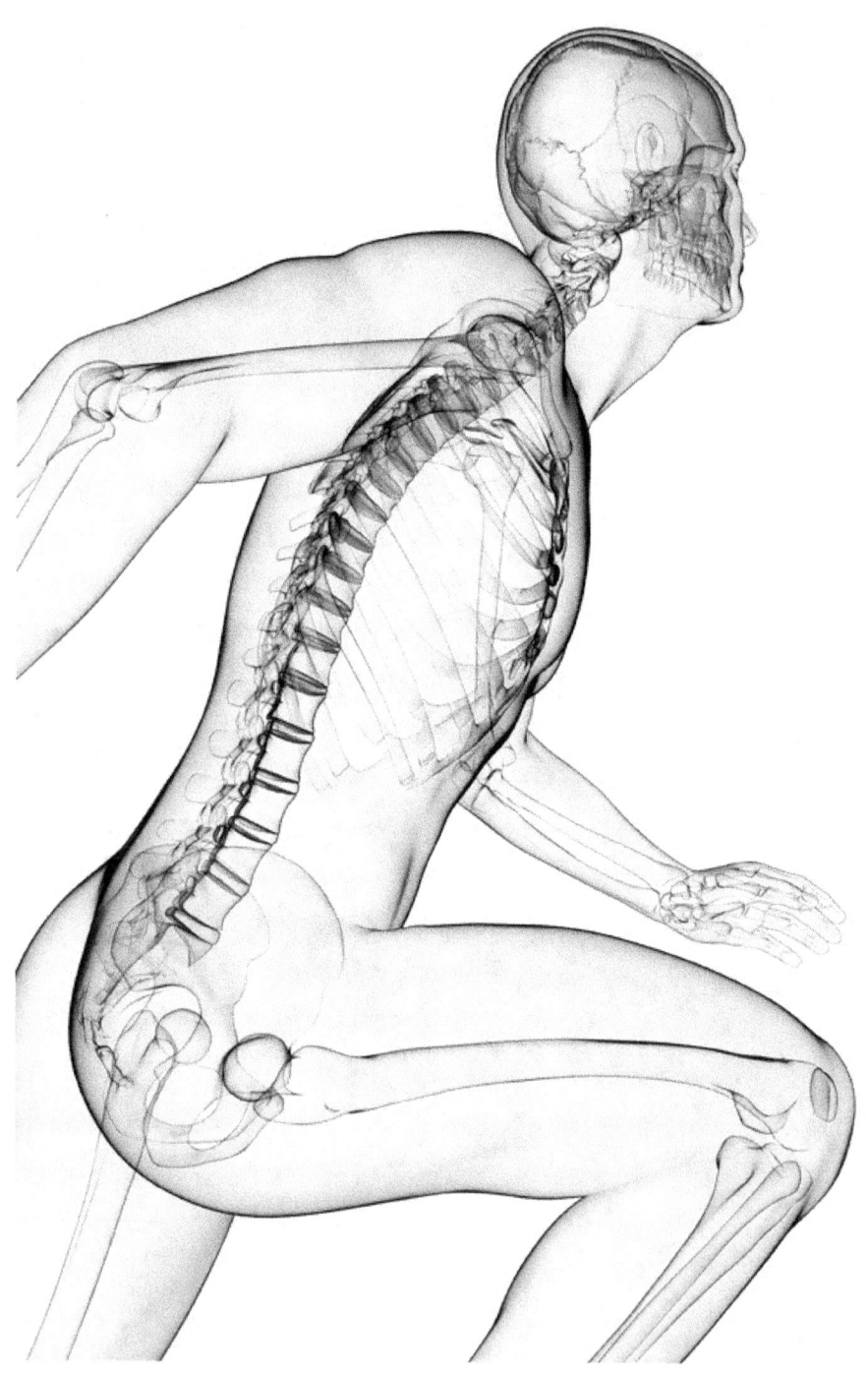

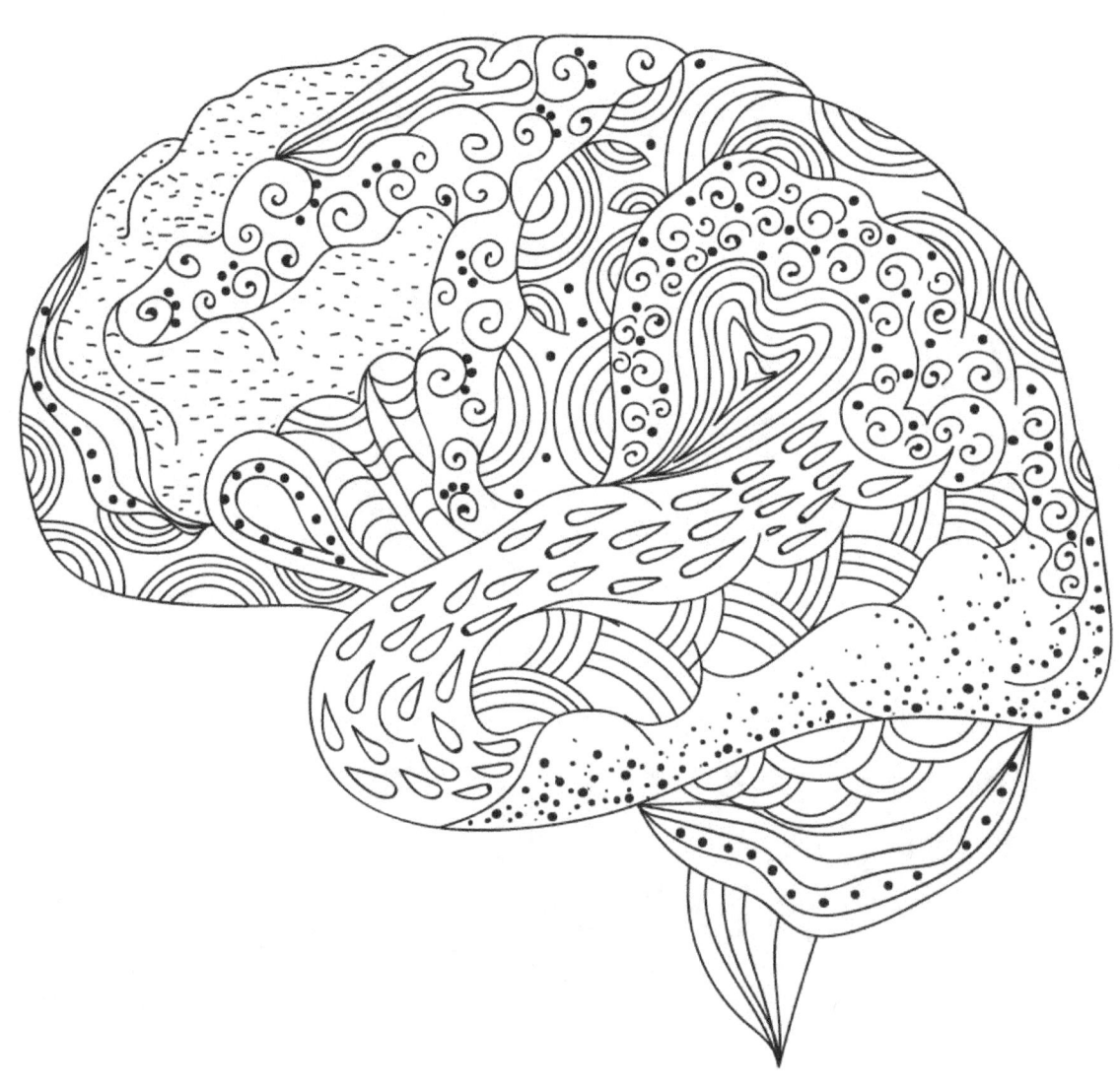

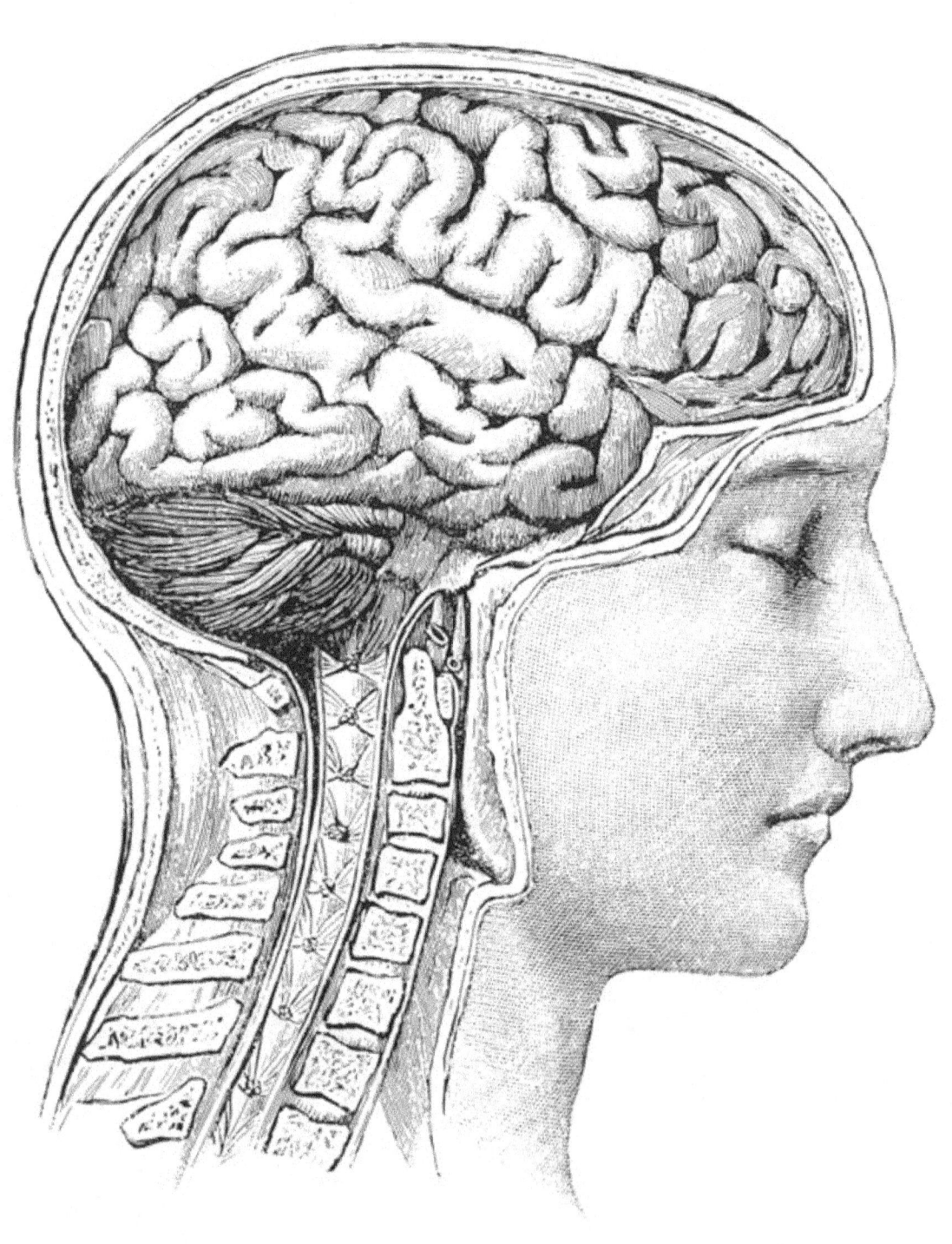

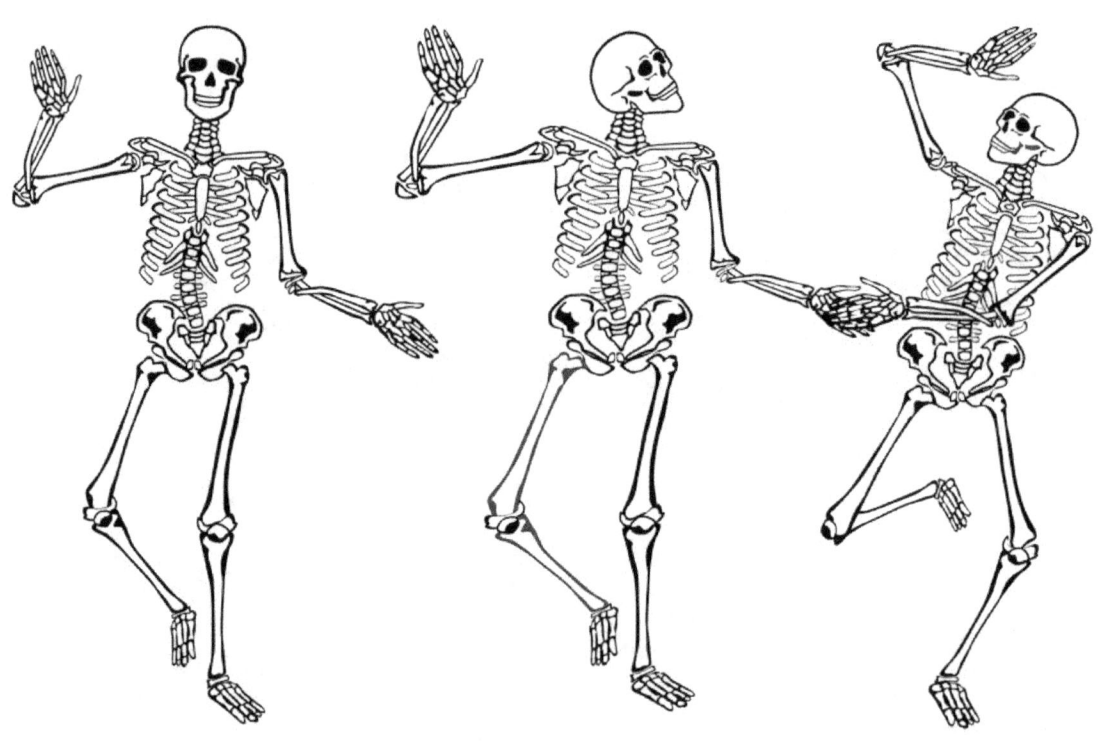

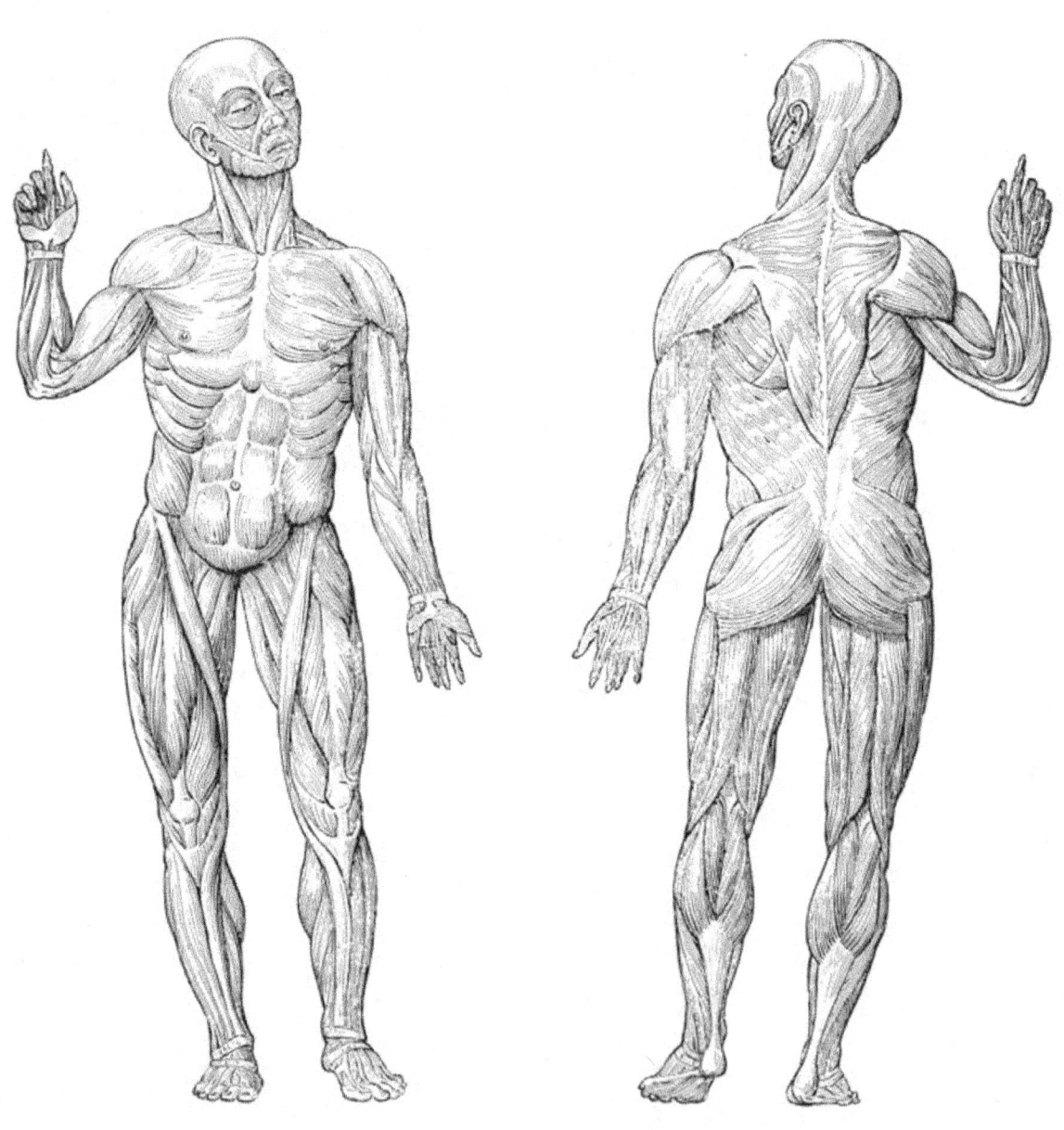

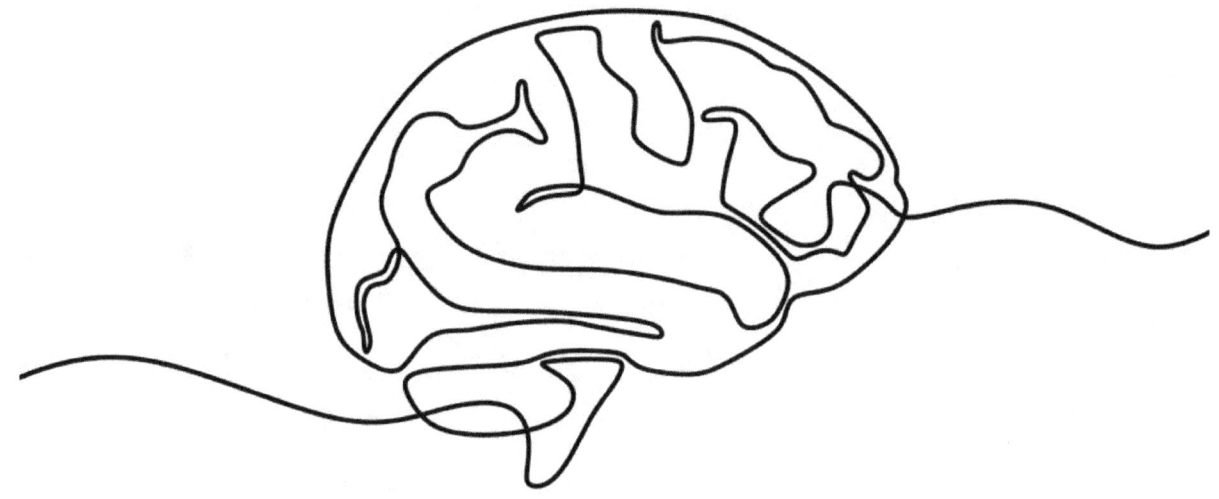

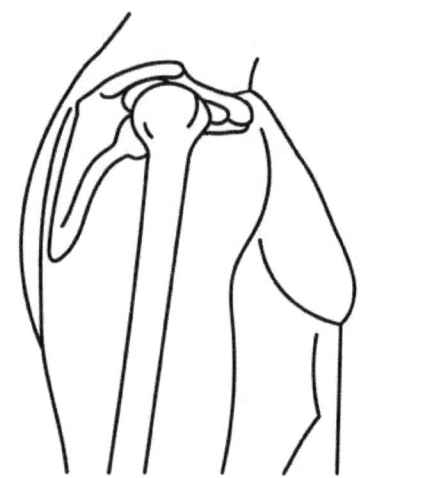
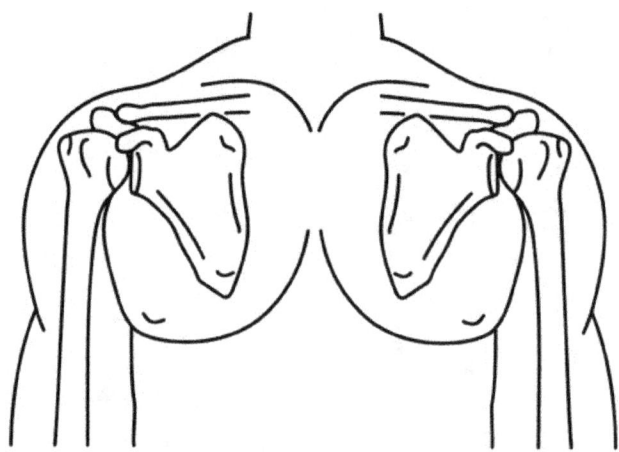

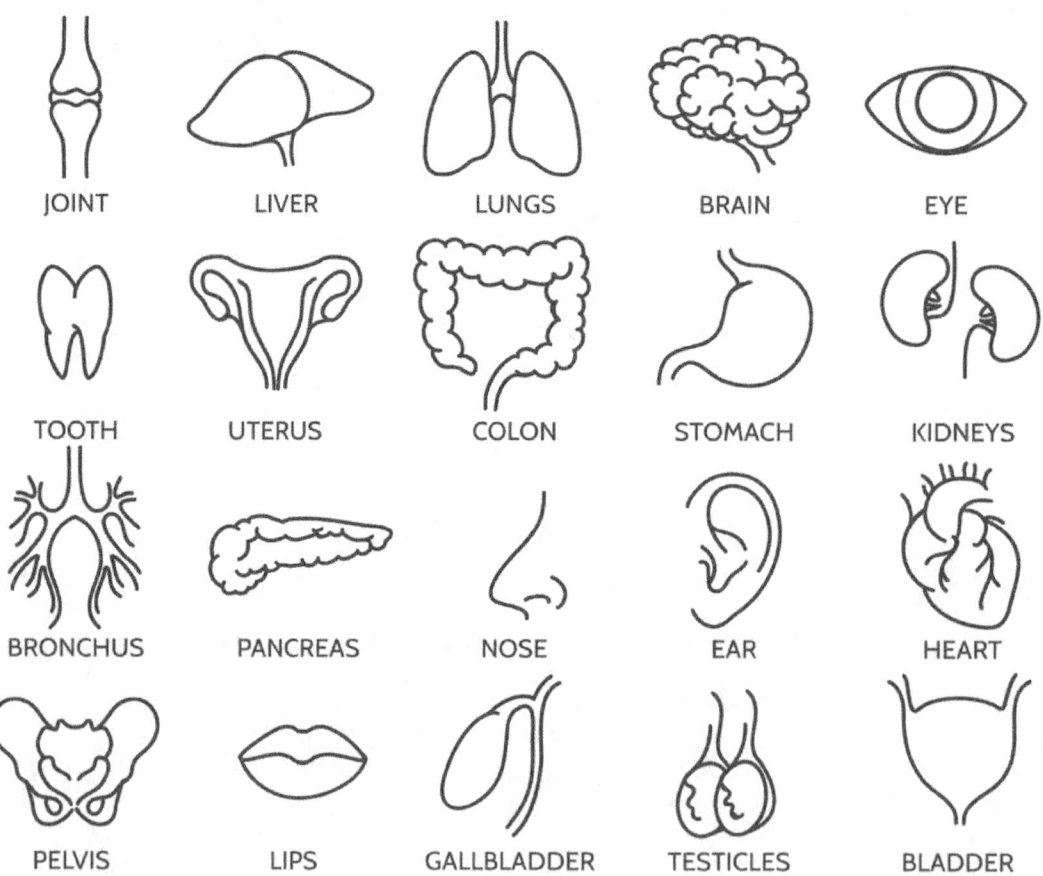